TEST YOUR KNOWLEDGE
MCQs
THE PATIENT WITH AN ENDOCRINE DISORDER

TEST YOUR KNOWLEDGE
MCQs
THE PATIENT WITH AN ENDOCRINE DISORDER

Grainne Anthony, SRN, RCNT, DipN (Lon), DipNEd (Lon), RNT
Senior Tutor

Victoria Belam, SRN, RNT
Senior Tutor

Judith Bristow, SRN, SCM DipN (Lon), RNT, DipEd
Senior Tutor

Josephine Humphrey, SRN, SCM, DipN(Lon), RCNT, DipNEd(Lon), RNT
Tutor

The Princess Alexandra School of Nursing
The London Hospital
London

Harper & Row, Publishers
London

Cambridge
Hagerstown
Philadelphia
New York

San Francisco
Mexico City
São Paulo
Sydney

Harper & Row Ltd
28 Tavistock Street
London WC2E 7PN

British Library Cataloguing in Publication Data

The patient with an endocrine disorder.—(Test your knowledge)
  1. Endocrine glands—Diseases
  I. Anthony, Grainne   II. Series
  616.4'0024613   RC649

  ISBN 0-06-318256-4

Typeset by Gedset Limited, Cheltenham.
Printed and bound by A Wheaton & Co Ltd, Exeter.

CONTENTS

FOREWORD

It gave me great pleasure indeed to be asked to write the foreword to this book.

The previous books in the series were written by four teachers of nursing working initially in the same school of nursing. The tradition is being carried on by Grainne Anthony, Josephine Humphrey, Judith Bristow and Victoria Belam, who are employed in the same school, and relate closely as professional colleagues, as well as being friends.

The aims of the series have not changed, that is to:

promote discussion
stimulate active learning
test understanding
aid self-assessment

The success of the series is shown not just by the sales of the books, but by the letters, comments and questions received by the authors from nurse learners and teachers.

Victoria, Judith, Josephine and Grainne have worked hard and consistently, with much gnashing of teeth and some tearing of hair, and I am sure you will agree that they have maintained the high standard set by the authors in the previous books.

E.R. Parker
MSc BA (Hons) SRN, RMN, SCM, RNT
1985

PREFACE

In 1981 the General Nursing Council for England and Wales published proposals for changes in the format of the multiple choice paper. As from January 1983, 30 of the questions have been unrelated and the other 30 related to stories about patients. The English National Board are again discussing changes in the examination system, and although the multiple choice paper may disappear sometime in the future we feel that these books still have a place as a learning tool.

The four previous authors, for various reasons, found it difficult to continue to meet to write the stories and asked us to take over the task to complete the series. We felt that the format had proved successful and so we have tried to follow it.

Multiple choice questions stimulate discussion in order to arrive at the answer, thus enhancing the problem-solving approach to patient-centred nursing. This aspect promotes learning as well as testing understanding. All the questions have been tried by our students and validated, and we would like to thank them all for their support and helpful suggestions.

We are also indebted to Pat Barry without whose superb secretarial skills we would never have been able to remain sane and produce this book.

How to use this book

Each question starts with a brief 'story' about the patient, followed by a series of related multiple choice questions.

It will be necessary to refer back to the story when selecting your answer, bearing in mind the individuality of the patient and the need to assess the effect that this may have on the care planned.

It is our belief that there is only one right answer to each question, and we have given our reasons for selecting this as the most appropriate answer in a section at the end of the book.

Example

Mrs Ellis   is an obese 68-year-old widow who lives alone in a council flat. She consulted her doctor because of failing sight and he discovered that she had glycosuria. She is admitted for assessment and during the admission interview she confides that she suffers from 'itching down below'.

1   Which of the following is the most likely cause of Mrs Ellis' pruritis? Infection by:
(a) *Streptococcus faecalis,*
(b) *Trichomonas vaginalis,*
(c) *Candida albicans,*
(d) *Escherichia coli.*

2   Which of the following is the purpose of the occupational therapist making a home visit with Mrs Ellis? To:
(a) identify the aids she needs,
(b) assess her activities of daily living,
(c) establish if she needs to be rehoused,
(d) determine her ability to cook for herself.

3   For which one of the following reasons will Mrs Ellis be advised against eating diabetic chocolate? It:
(a) raises blood glucose rapidly,
(b) raises blood glucose slowly,
(c) is carcinogenic,
(d) is fattening.

Answers to Example

1 (c) This fungus thrives in a
glucose medium and infection
causes itching.
2 (b) Assessment is necessary to
identify her needs.
3 (d) Diabetic chocolate contains
sorbitol.

Mrs Margaret James aged 52 years, is the wife of a successful businessman. Her husband travels extensively and her two children are both married and busy raising their own families. Recently she consulted her GP complaining of depression, irregular menstruation, dyspareunia and hot flushes. Her obvious embarrassment at discussing such personal problems led her doctor to refer her to a menopause clinic.

1   Which one of the following is the correct definition of the menopause?
    (a) the phase during which reproductive function ceases,
    (b) absence of menses for one year,
    (c) progressive ovarian failure,
    (d) the last menstrual bleed.

2   Which of the following is the most probable reason for Mrs James' depression?
    (a) loneliness and feelings of uselessness,
    (b) physical symptoms of the climacteric,
    (c) loss of ovarian function,
    (d) loss of libido.

3   Which of the following will be most helpful to Mrs James when she complains of hot flushes?
    (a) 'It's normal at your age and will gradually stop.'
    (b) 'They can be reduced by avoiding alcohol and keeping cool.'
    (c) 'Your vascular system is responding to hormonal imbalances.'
    (d) 'If you concentrate on other things they won't be so severe.'

4   Which of the following is the most probable reason for Mrs James' dyspareunia?
    (a) clumsy coitus,
    (b) loss of libido,
    (c) vaginal infection,
    (d) diminished vaginal secretions.

5   Which of the following will be the most help to Mrs James at the climacteric?
    (a) the opportunity to discuss her symptoms,
    (b) encouragement to occupy her time,
    (c) hormonal replacement therapy,
    (d) vitamin B_6 supplements.

6   For which of the following reasons is prolonged oestrogen therapy contra-
    indicated? There is an increased risk of:
    (a) deep-vein thrombosis,
    (b) cirrhosis of the liver,
    (c) carcinoma of the breast,
    (d) carcinoma of the endometrium.

7   Which one of the following is the main role of the nurse specialist in a
    menopause clinic?
    (a) adviser,
    (b) educator,
    (c) counsellor,
    (d) therapist.

8   Which of the following conditions will Mrs James be exposed to following
    the menopause?
    (a) depression,
    (b) osteoporosis,
    (c) carcinoma of the uterus,
    (d) maturity onset diabetes.

David Sutton   is a 17-year-old member of the sixth form at school. He
enjoys reading and playing football. He has recently been diagnosed as having
diabetes mellitus which is now controlled by diet and insulin.

1   Which one of the following should David be advised to increase in his diet?
    (a) water,
    (b) fibre,
    (c) protein,
    (d) unsaturated fat.

2   For which one of the following reasons should David rotate his injection
    sites? To avoid:
    (a) bruising,
    (b) infection,
    (c) fibrosed tissue,
    (d) painful swelling.

3   Which of the following should David be advised to avoid?
    (a) drinking alcohol,
    (b) walking barefoot,

(c) wearing contact lenses,
(d) eating all forms of sugar.

4   Which one of the following fluids may David drink whenever he desires?
    (a) skimmed milk,
    (b) black coffee,
    (c) ginger beer,
    (d) fruit juice.

5   Which one of the following answers will be given when David asks 'Do I
    have to pay for the insulin and syringe?'
        (a) 'All prescribed items are free',
        (b) 'You need to pay for all prescribed items,'
        (c) 'You need to pay for prescribed diabetic items,'
        (d) 'You only pay for prescribed nondiabetic items.'

Mrs Prudence Whittaker   aged 68 years, attended her GP's surgery
complaining of vulval pruritis and increasing lassitude. The doctor arranged
to test her urine, which showed 2% sugar, and sent a blood sample to the local
hospital for estimation of serum glucose. He referred her to a consultant
physician with suspected diabetes mellitus.

1   From which of the following may Mrs Whittaker also suffer?
    (a) polyuria, weight loss,
    (b) weight loss, dysuria,
    (c) obesity, polyuria,
    (d) dysuria, obesity.

2   For which one of the following reasons is it important to explain to Mrs
    Whittaker what diabetes mellitus is?
    (a) it is her body therefore she needs to know,
    (b) to help her recognize the complications,
    (c) understanding helps bring co-operation,
    (d) so that she understands her diet.

3   Which one of the following people should Mrs Whittaker consult, as well
    as the doctor, each time she attends out-patients? The:
    (a) opthalmologist,
    (b) social worker,
    (c) chiropodist,
    (d) dietician.

4   Which of the following is the most appropriate response to give Mrs
     Whittaker when she asks if she can still drink alcohol?
     (a) avoid beer, but gin and whisky are free of carbohydrate,
     (b) yes, within her calorie and carbohydrate allowance,
     (c) yes, provided it is dry wine or sherry,
     (d) she should avoid all alcohol.

Mr Maurice Kenney   aged 56 years, is admitted to the ward for a below-
knee amputation. He has been a diabetic for 40 years and has, during that
time, remained well. For the last 18 months he has had a discharging ulcer on
his right big toe which has failed to respond to medical treatment.

1   Which one of the following is the most likely predisposing factor of Mr
     Kenney's ulcer?
     (a) atherosclerosis,
     (b) arteriosclerosis,
     (c) peripheral neuritis,
     (d) nutritional neuritis.

2   Which of the following is the most appropriate response to give a junior
     nurse who asks why Mr Kenney is having a below-knee amputation for a
     discharging toe? It:
     (a) is easier to fit a prosthesis,
     (b) is an easier operation to perform,
     (c) means that he will not need any more surgery,
     (d) increases the chances of good healing.

3   Which of the following will play the most important part in the immediate
     preparation for surgery?
     (a) the physiotherapist,
     (b) a successful amputee,
     (c) the prosthetic engineer,
     (d) the occupational therapist.

4   Which of the following is essential for Mr Kenney to learn as soon as
     possible?
     (a) use of elbow crutches,
     (b) his centre of gravity,
     (c) how his new prosthesis works,
     (d) how to transfer from bed to wheelchair.

Mrs Jennings   is a recently widowed 58-year-old lady. She has been admitted for a subtotal thyroidectomy. During surgery considerable difficulty was experienced in mobilizing a large retrosternal extension of the right lobe, which resulted in a small haemorrhage. Haemostasis was achieved and the wound closed with skin clips. Two vacuum drains were inserted. On return to the ward she is conscious and vital signs are stable within normal limits. A transfusion of AB negative blood is in progress.

1   To which one of the following blood groups does Mrs Jennings belong?
 (a) A negative,
 (b) B negative,
 (c) AB positive,
 (d) O positive.

2   Which of the following specific areas must be observed by the nurse?
 (a) the wound,
 (b) the nape of her neck,
 (c) her swallowing reflex,
 (d) her lips and nail beds.

3   Of which of the following will Mrs Jennings complain if she has a haemorrhage?
 (a) nausea and sweating,
 (b) a choking sensation,
 (c) a feeling of faintness,
 (d) feeling cold and clammy.

4   Which one of the following would be an indication that Mrs Jennings was bleeding into the tissues?
 (a) cyanosis,
 (b) dyspnoea,
 (c) dysphagia,
 (d) air hunger.

5   Which of the following is the most appropriate action to take when Mrs Jennings suddenly complains of shortness of breath? Notify the doctor and:
 (a) remove skin clips,
 (b) administer humidified oxygen,
 (c) prepare tracheostomy equipment,
 (d) sit her in the orthopnoeic position.

6   Which one of the following types of haemorrhage has Mrs Jennings
    experienced?
    (a) primary,
    (b) secondary,
    (c) tertiary,
    (d) reactionary.

Mrs Emma Blake   aged 60 years, has been taking steroid therapy for
the last 5 years. Recently she became concerned because of backache and
excessive facial hair. She has been admitted to your ward for assessment of
her condition.

1   Which one of the following is most likely to be found when testing Mrs
    Blake's urine?
    (a) blood,
    (b) glucose,
    (c) ketones,
    (d) protein.

2   Which of the following is most appropriate when administering Mrs
    Blake's steroids? The tablets should be:
    (a) effervescent,
    (b) enteric coated,
    (c) swallowed with milk,
    (d) administered after food.

3   Which one of the following would be the most likely cause of Mrs Blake's
    backache?
    (a) osteochondritis,
    (b) osteoarthrosis,
    (c) osteoporosis,
    (d) osteomyelitis.

4   Which one of the following should you advise when Mrs Blake complains
    about her excessive facial hair?
    (a) electrolysis,
    (b) use facial wax,
    (c) shave when necessary,
    (d) try a cream depilatory.

5   Which of the following is the most important advice to give before Mrs
    Blake is discharged? To:
    (a) weigh herself weekly,
    (b) eat a salt-free diet,
    (c) test her urine twice daily,
    (d) avoid people with colds.

Debbie Frances   is a 30-year-old air hostess. Investigations 10 weeks ago
confirmed a diagnosis of hyperthyroidism. She has now been admitted to your
ward for a partial thyroidectomy.

1   Which one of the following would reduce the vascularity of Debbie's
    thyroid gland?
    (a) carbimazole,
    (b) propranolol,
    (c) potassium iodide,
    (d) radioactive iodine.

2   Which one of the following must be performed before Debbie's operation?
    (a) thyroid scan,
    (b) ophthalmoscopy,
    (c) serum calcium levels,
    (d) examination of her vocal cords.

3   Which of the following observations is most important in the detection of
    thyroid crisis?
    (a) temperature,
    (b) respirations,
    (c) blood pressure,
    (d) muscle twitching.

4   On which of the following days should Debbie's clips be removed? The:
    (a) 3rd-5th day,
    (b) 5th-7th day,
    (c) 7th-9th day,
    (d) 9th-11th day.

5   Which one of the following should be suspected if Debbie complained of a
    hoarse voice persisting for more than 4 days?
    (a) laryngitis,
    (b) pharyngeal oedema,

(c) damage to the vocal cords,
(d) injury of a recurrent laryngeal nerve.

6   Which of the following is the most apppropriate information to give
    Debbie when she is discharged?
    (a) 'Use unperfumed soap to avoid irritation of your scar.'
    (b) 'Massage lanolin on your scar to keep the skin supple.'
    (c) 'Cover the scar with a dressing until it is completely healed.'
    (d) 'Spray the scar with a clear plastic dressing to keep it waterproof.'

7   Which one of the following responses is most appropriate when Debbie
    expresses concern about the cosmetic effect of surgery on her neck? The
    scar:
    (a) may fade eventually,
    (b) follows a skin fold,
    (c) can always be covered up,
    (d) is less obtrusive than her swollen neck.

Mr Ross   is a 68-year-old diabetic who has been in hospital for treatment of
a deep ulcer on his left heel, which has now healed. The ulcer resulted from
wearing a new pair of shoes on a day trip with the pensioners' club. Mr Ross has
clawing of the toes and calluses on the soles of both feet.

1   By which one of the following processes will Mr Ross' ulcer have healed?
    (a) fibrosis,
    (b) granulation,
    (c) first intention,
    (d) second intention.

2   Which of the following precautions should Mr Ross take before washing
    his feet?
    (a) run the cold water first,
    (b) test the water with his hand,
    (c) test the water with his elbow,
    (d) run the cold and hot water together.

3   Which of the following should Mr Ross avoid using?
    (a) bed socks,
    (b) a heat pad,
    (c) heavy blankets,
    (d) a hot water bottle.

4   Which of the following is the reason for the clawing of Mr Ross' toes?
    (a) badly fitting shoes,
    (b) recurrent plantar ulcers,
    (c) lack of sensation in the toes,
    (d) paralysis of the small muscles of the feet.

5   Which of the following is the cause of the calluses on Mr Ross' feet?
    Hyperkeratosis due to:
    (a) deformity of the toes,
    (b) badly fitting shoes,
    (c) diabetes mellitus,
    (d) lack of foot care.

6   Which one of the following is the safe method for Mr Ross to treat the
    calluses on his feet? Use of a:
    (a) callus pad,
    (b) pumice stone,
    (c) corn plaster,
    (d) chemical keratolytic.

7   Which one of the following procedures should Mr Ross follow when he
    buys new shoes?
    (a) insert shoe trees when not in use,
    (b) wear them around the house for a couple of days,
    (c) wear them for gradually increasing periods of time,
    (d) wear them for 2 hour periods and inspect his feet after each wear.

Mrs Julia Craven   aged 25 years, is admitted to your ward for investigations of thyrotoxicosis.

1   Which one of the following positions in the ward would be most
    appropriate for Mrs Craven?
    (a) close to the toilet area in case she has diarrhoea,
    (b) near the nurses' station for observation,
    (c) in a side room to prevent disturbance,
    (d) next to a window to keep her cool.

2   Of which of the following problems may Mrs Craven complain?
    (a) exophthalmos, anorexia, weight loss,
    (b) amenorrhoea, sweating, palpitations,
    (c) weight loss, irritability, dysphagia,
    (d) irritability, menorrhagia, exophthalmos.

3   Which one of the following responses would be most appropriate when Mrs Craven expresses concern about her exophthalmos? That it:
(a) may improve following treatment,
(b) will disappear eventually,
(c) is irreversible,
(d) is treatable.

4   Which of the following beverages is most suitable for Mrs Craven?
(a) tea,
(b) coffee,
(c) coca cola,
(d) carbonated water.

5   Which of the following is most important when monitoring Mrs Craven's condition?
(a) blood pressure,
(b) urine output,
(c) temperature,
(d) weight.

6   Which one of the following should be performed to help diagnose Mrs Craven's condition?
(a) ophthalmoscopy,
(b) 24-hour urine collection,
(c) observation of sleeping pulse,
(d) examination of the vocal cords.

7   Which one of the following drugs should improve Mrs Craven's toxic state?
(a) diazepam,
(b) carbimazole,
(c) Lugol's iodine,
(d) potassium iodide.

Constance Smith   is a 20-year-old typist. She visited her family doctor because she was very concerned that her 'body was changing', and she complained of headaches and muscular weakness. She was found to be hypertensive and an appointment was made for her to visit the endocrinologist at the City Hospital for investigations of Cushing's disease.

1   Which of the following may be found when observing Constance?
(a) loss of limb muscle, facial plethora, central obesity,

(b) facial plethora, loss of limb muscle, weight loss,
(c) thick skin, central obesity, hirsutism,
(d) weight loss, hirsutism, thick skin.

2   Which of the following may be found when observing Constance's skin?
   (a) pruritis, striae, acne,
   (b) bruising, acne, striae,
   (c) acne, urticaria, pruritis,
   (d) striae, bruising, urticaria.

3   For which one of the following reasons will Constance develop excessive body hair? Excess:
   (a) androgen,
   (b) oestrogen,
   (c) progesterone,
   (d) glucocorticoids.

4   Which of the following will the doctor ask Constance to do in order to assess her muscle weakness? To:
   (a) lift some weights,
   (b) get up from the chair,
   (c) run up and down on the spot,
   (d) bend down and touch her toes.

5   Which one of the following is the reason for her muscle weakness?
   (a) hypokalaemia,
   (b) hyponatraemia,
   (c) hypermyotonia,
   (d) hypercalcaemia.

6   Which of the following explains Constance's hypertension? The:
   (a) very rapid weight gain,
   (b) excess androgen hormones,
   (c) catabolic effect of hydrocortisone,
   (d) sodium-retaining effect of cortisol.

Miss Evelyn Gladwell   aged 40 years, is an artist and lives alone. Her sister from Canada visited her for a holiday and was amazed how Evelyn had changed in appearance. She encouraged her to visit her doctor who diagnosed myxoedema. She is now in hospital for investigations and treatment.

1   Which of the following recordings should you expect from Miss
    Gladwell's observations?
    (a) bradycardia and hypothermia,
    (b) tachypnoea and hypotension,
    (c) bradycardia and hypertension,
    (d) hypothermia and hypertension.

2   Which of the following may be observed when nursing Miss Gladwell?
    (a) polyuria, coarse skin, lethargy,
    (b) coarse skin, lethargy, sparse hair,
    (c) sparse hair, polyuria, weight loss,
    (d) lethargy, weight loss, constipation.

3   Which one of the following should be used to provide Miss Gladwell with
    extra comfort?
    (a) offer her a bedpan hourly,
    (b) give her extra blankets,
    (c) give warm milky drinks,
    (d) provide a heat pad.

4   For which one of the following reasons will Miss Gladwell complain of
    tingling sensations in her hands?
    (a) tennis elbow,
    (b) ulnar neuritis,
    (c) frozen shoulder syndrome,
    (d) median nerve compression.

5   Which of the following is the appropriate advice to give Miss Gladwell
    before she is discharged home?
    (a) stress that treatment is for life,
    (b) sleep in the semi-recumbent position,
    (c) always carry your drug card with you,
    (d) keep appointments for your weekly blood tests.

6   Which one of the following complications may Miss Gladwell develop if
    she does not have treatment?
    (a) coma,
    (b) chloasma,
    (c) catalepsy,
    (d) cretinism.

Mrs Ruth Coates   a widow aged 38 years, is admitted to a surgical ward for
a bilateral adrenalectomy because of adrenocortical hyperplasia.

1   Which one of the following diets will Mrs Coates most likely be prescribed?
    (a) reducing,
    (b) salt free,
    (c) high protein,
    (d) fluid restriction.

2   Which one of the following may be administered intravenously to Mrs
    Coates preoperatively?
    (a) potassium chloride,
    (b) calcium gluconate,
    (c) sodium chloride,
    (d) sodium lactate.

3   Which one of the following problems must the nurse report immediately
    when nursing Mrs Coates postoperatively?
    (a) loin pain,
    (b) bradycardia,
    (c) hypotension,
    (d) tingling of hands.

4   Which of the following are monitored regularly and influence the amount
    of corticoids given?
    (a) sodium, potassium, glucose,
    (b) glucose, chloride, potassium,
    (c) potassium, bicarbonate, sodium,
    (d) bicarbonate, glucose, chloride.

5   Which one of the following actions is most important before Mrs Coates
    begins to be mobilized?
    (a) remove the wound drain,
    (b) elevate the head of the bed,
    (c) apply anti-embolic stockings,
    (d) discontinue intravenous therapy.

Mrs Reeves   is a 43-year-old housewife who recently found a lump in her
left breast. It was diagnosed as being stage-one carcinoma and she has had a
left simple mastectomy. She will have a course of radiotherapy to start 6
weeks after her operation.

1   Which of the following is the percentage of breast lumps which are found
    to be malignant?
    (a) 10%,
    (b) 25%,
    (c) 50%,
    (d) 75%.

2   Which of the following describes simple mastectomy? Removal of:
    (a) breast tissue only,
    (b) breast tissue, underlying muscle,
    (c) breast tissue and axillary lymph nodes,
    (d) breast tissue and underlying lymph nodes.

3   For which of the following reasons will Mrs Reeve's arm be supported on a
    pillow following surgery? So that it is:
    (a) in a comfortable position,
    (b) above the level of the right atrium,
    (c) in a position to allow venous return,
    (d) above the level of the left ventricle.

4   For which of the following reasons will Mrs Reeves be discouraged from
    exercising her arm until the physiotherapist is present? Because uncon-
    trolled exercise may result in:
    (a) haemorrhage,
    (b) excessive scar tissue,
    (c) delayed wound healing,
    (d) necrosis of the wound edges.

5   Which of the following will enable Mrs Reeves to use a temporary
    prosthesis in the first weeks following surgery? Having:
    (a) a front-opening bra,
    (b) a bra made to measure,
    (c) a pocket sewn into a new bra,
    (d) a pocket sewn into an old bra.

6   Which of the following is the correct response when Mrs Reeves expresses
    concern about the effects of radiotherapy on her skin?
    (a) you can expect a slight skin reaction,
    (b) if you follow instructions you will have no problems,
    (c) radiation burns are common with this type of treatment,
    (d) your skin will be red and sore for the duration of the treatment.

Jennifer and **Tim Mills**   have been married for 5 years. They delayed starting a family for 3 years for financial reasons, during which time Jennifer took a contraceptive pill. Now they have consulted their doctor who has referred them to an infertility clinic.

1   Which one of the following best defines infertility? Failure to conceive following unprotected coitus for:
(a) 2 years,
(b) 18 months,
(c) 1 year,
(d) 6 months.

2   Which one of the following is the most probable cause of Jennifer and Tim's infertility?
(a) anxiety,
(b) a low sperm count,
(c) disordered ovulation,
(d) pelvic inflammatory disease.

3   Which one of the following tests is most reliable to assess Jennifer's ovulation? A:
(a) continuous record of basal body temperature to assess the time of ovulation,
(b) cervical smear to assess the effect of progesterone on the epithelium,
(c) measurement of serial plasma progesterone levels to assess luteal function,
(d) collection of cervical mucus to assess penetrability by sperm.

4   In which one of the following ways should the nurse advise Tim and Jennifer to obtain a sample of semen for analysis? By:
(a) masturbation,
(b) coitus interuptus,
(c) post-coital urine specimen,
(d) post-coital cervical smear.

5   During which one of the following time periods should Jennifer and Tim be advised to have coitus?·
(a) during the mid-cycle period,
(b) once ovulation has occurred,
(c) continuously throughout the menstrual cycle,
(d) immediately the menstrual flow has stopped until it starts again.

6 Which one of the following is the most appropriate way to help Jennifer
   and Tim if their tests prove inconclusive?
   (a) referral to an adoption agency,
   (b) reassurance that parenthood is possible,
   (c) encouragement to continue trying to conceive,
   (d) counselling to help them accept their infertility.

Mrs Mary West   aged 34 years, is recovering from a partial thyroidectomy
performed 18 hours ago. During the early hours of the morning she became
hyperpyrexial and disorientated. A thyroid crisis was diagnosed.

1 Which of the following symptoms may Mrs West have in addition to
   hyperpyrexia?
   (a) hypertension, diarrhoea, restlessness,
   (b) tachycardia, restlessness, diarrhoea,
   (c) vomiting, hypertension, restlessness,
   (d) restlessness, tachycardia, vomiting.

2 Which of the following drugs is most appropriate to reduce Mrs West's
   pyrexia?
   (a) aspirin,
   (b) diazepam,
   (c) carbimazole,
   (d) chlorpromazine.

3 For which of the following reasons is it most important for Mrs West to
   have an intravenous infusion? To ensure a:
   (a) regular fluid intake,
   (b) continuous glucose infusion,
   (c) reduction in body temperature,
   (d) route for the administration of drugs.

4 Which of the following antithyroid drugs is most likely to be given to Mrs
   West?
   (a) carbimazole,
   (b) Lugol's iodine,
   (c) propylthiouracil,
   (d) potassium iodide.

Mark Springer   is 24 years old and has been diabetic for 6 years. He is admitted to hospital for re-assessment of his diabetes following a severe hypoglycaemic attack which he did not recognize. During the admission interview it emerges that he has recently had several mild hypoglycaemic attacks and that he occasionally exchanges a glass of whisky for part of his lunchtime carbohydrate allowance.

1   Which one of the following is the first action the nurse should take if she suspects that Mark is having a hypoglycaemic attack?
(a) call the doctor,
(b) give him a sweet drink,
(c) prepare a glucagon injection,
(d) measure his blood glucose levels.

2   Which one of the following contains 10 g of glucose?
(a) two teaspoons of sugar,
(b) four teaspoons of sugar,
(c) 50 ml of orange juice,
(d) 200 ml of orange juice.

3   Which of the following is the correct response when Mark asks why he should not drink whisky? Because it:
(a) causes hyperglycaemia,
(b) reduces manual dexterity,
(c) interferes with awareness,
(d) predisposes to hypoglycaemia.

4   Which one of the following will ensure that Mark recognizes a hypogly-caemic attack in future?
(a) enable him to experience an attack,
(b) explain the symptoms of hypoglycaemia,
(c) explain the factors that cause hypoglycaemia,
(d) enable him to discuss how he felt during his last attack.

5   Which one of the following causes sweating and palpitations during an hypoglycaemic attack?
(a) insulin lack,
(b) glucagon production,
(c) adrenaline stimulation,
(d) glucocorticoid secretion.

Gareth Morgan   a 15-year-old schoolboy, has recently been diagnosed as having diabetes mellitus. He is preparing for 'O' level examinations and is a star in the school rugby team.

1   Which of the following is the aim of Gareth's care? To:
    (a) improve his fat metabolism,
    (b) maintain a normal life style,
    (c) improve carbohydrate metabolism,
    (d) maintain normal blood glucose levels.

2   Which of the following is the first step in teaching Gareth about his diabetes?
    (a) determine his knowledge of normal physiology,
    (b) determine his knowledge of diabetes,
    (c) explain what diabetes mellitus is,
    (d) explain carbohydrate metabolism.

3   For which one of the following reasons will Gareth's energy requirements be greater than those of an adult? Because his intake must meet the demands of:
    (a) playing rugby with the school team,
    (b) replacement of glucose stores,
    (c) preparing for examinations,
    (d) adolescent growth.

4   For which one of the following reasons should Gareth have a snack at bedtime? To:
    (a) prevent hypoglycaemia whilst sleeping,
    (b) maintain normal blood glucose levels,
    (c) provide energy in the early morning,
    (d) ensure normal metabolism at night.

5   For which one of the following reasons will Gareth be advised to rotate his injection sites? Because constant use of one site will lead to:
    (a) infection,
    (b) inflammation,
    (c) abscess formation,
    (d) reduced absorption.

6   For which one of the following reasons must Gareth be taught not to handle the Clinitest tablets? It may:
    (a) discolour the skin,

(b) cause a caustic burn,
(c) give a false positive,
(d) decrease the sensitivity of the tablet.

7   Which one of the following actions should Gareth take on the days he
    plays rugby?
    (a) increase his insulin dose,
    (b) decrease his insulin dose,
    (c) increase his energy intake,
    (d) decrease his energy intake.

Mr John Wellington   aged 47 years, an area sales manager, has been
admitted for a hypophysectomy. He was diagnosed 2 years ago as having
acromegaly and had been treated medically with little effect. The symptoms
were having an increasing effect on his life style and work performance.

1   Which one of the following drugs would have been given to Mr Wellington
    to try and control his symptoms?
    (a) bromocriptine,
    (b) benzonatate,
    (c) bromhexine,
    (d) benzocaine.

2   Which of the following signs and symptoms are those of acromegaly?
    (a) headache, bitemporal hemianopia, paraesthesia of fingers,
    (b) bilateral anosmia, paraesthesia of fingers, headache,
    (c) dysarthria, headache, nystagmus,
    (d) nystagmus, dysphasia, headache.

3   Which of the following best explains hypophysectomy? It is the surgical
    removal of the:
    (a) pituitary gland,
    (b) hypothalamus,
    (c) thymus gland,
    (d) epiphysis.

4   Which one of the following drugs will Mr Wellington require with his
    premedication?
    (a) hydrocortisone,
    (b) dexamethasone,

(c) vasopressin,
(d) thyroxine.

5   Which of the following are most important when observing Mr Wellington after surgery?
(a) blood pressure, nasal discharge, urine output,
(b) blood pressure, aural discharge, urine output,
(c) limb movement, pulse, fluid intake,
(d) pupil action, pulse, fluid intake.

6   Which one of the following should the nurse expect when testing Mr Wellington's urine postoperatively?
(a) high specific gravity, pale in colour,
(b) high specific gravity, dark in colour,
(c) low specific gravity, pale in colour,
(d) low specific gravity, dark in colour.

Mr Victor Bussolino   aged 68 years, a widower, who has been a diabetic for the last 18 years is now complaining of severe pain in his left foot. He has been admitted for consideration of a below-knee amputation following a diagnosis of 'dry' gangrene. His niece, who is very anxious about the possibility of surgery, accompanies him to the ward.

1   Which of the following explanations best describes dry gangrene?
(a) infection by anaerobic organisms,
(b) infection by aerobic organisms,
(c) severe arterial insufficiency,
(d) severe venous insufficiency.

2   Which of the following is most important to note when taking his admission history?
(a) if he uses a hearing aid,
(b) whether he wears dentures,
(c) if he experiences nocturia,
(d) whether he appears to see normally.

3   Which of the following should form part of the nursing management of Mr Bussolino?
(a) mobilize within his capabilities,
(b) up for toilet purposes only,
(c) complete bed rest,
(d) barrier nursing.

4   Which of the following nursing actions is the most appropriate when dealing with Mr Bussolino's gangrenous foot?
(a) soak twice daily in potassium permanganate solution,
(b) dress daily with eusol and liquid paraffin,
(c) apply a dry dressing and bandage,
(d) leave exposed.

5   Which one of the following nursing actions is the most effective measure in helping to relieve the severe pain in his foot?
(a) provide a heat pad,
(b) elevate the foot of the bed,
(c) encourage him to hang the foot out of the bed,
(d) use a bed cradle to relieve the weight of the bed clothes.

6   Which one of the following drugs is Mr Bussolino likely to have been taking to help control his diabetes?
(a) chlorpheniramine,
(b) chlorpropramide,
(c) chlormethiazole,
(d) chlorambucil.

7   Which one of the following investigations will be necessary pre-operatively? Serum:
(a) globulin,
(b) albumin,
(c) calcium,
(d) lipids.

8   Which one of the following is most important before Mr Bussolino's surgery?
(a) electrocardiogram,
(b) angiography,
(c) chest X-ray,
(d) venogram.

9   Which of the following is most important for the nurse to monitor?
(a) pulse,
(b) respiration,
(c) temperature,
(d) blood pressure.

Miss Rita Walsh   aged 20 years, is admitted to a medical ward for investigations and treatment of Addison's disease.

1   Of which of the following problems is Rita most likely to complain?
(a) tiredness, bruising, weight loss,
(b) bruising, stretch marks, tiredness,
(c) weight loss, tiredness, darkened skin areas,
(d) darkened skin areas, tiredness, stretch marks.

2   Which one of the following is the main aim of Rita's nursing care? To prevent:
(a) haemorrhage,
(b) weight loss,
(c) depression,
(d) infection.

3   Which of the following is the most appropriate position in the ward for Rita?
(a) by the nurses' station,
(b) near the toilets,
(c) near the window,
(d) in a side room.

4   Which one of the following problems should you particularly observe when nursing Rita?
(a) cyanosis,
(b) faintness,
(c) photophobia,
(d) haemorrhage.

5   Which one of the following systolic blood pressure readings do you expect Rita to have?
(a) 90 mmHg,
(b) 110 mmHg,
(c) 130 mmHg,
(d) 150 mmHg.

6   Which of the following is the appropriate response when Rita asks 'Will my skin stay this colour for ever?'
(a) it will fade in about 18 months,
(b) it will disappear after treatment,
(c) the dermatologist has been contacted,
(d) the skilful use of cosmetics will conceal it.

7   Which of the following is Rita likely to develop if untreated?
    (a) hypertension and dehydration,
    (b) hypotension and dehydration,
    (c) hypertension and oedema,
    (d) hypotension and oedema.

8   Which one of the following should be the first line of treatment for Rita?
    (a) plasmaphoresis,
    (b) haemodialysis,
    (c) radiotherapy,
    (d) chemotherapy.

Mrs Sylvia Thorn   aged 50 years, has had a lump in her neck for many years. Recently she has noticed that she perspires excessively, cannot tolerate warm weather, suffers from palpitations, and is in a permanent state of anxiety and irritability. She satisfied herself that these symptoms were due to the menopause, but her husband was so concerned that he insisted she saw her doctor, who has requested her admission to hospital for further investigations for thyrotoxicosis.

1   Which of the following will be evident on examination of 10 ml of Mrs Thorn's clotted blood? A:
    (a) high level of tetra-iodothyronine,
    (b) high level of tri-iodothyronine,
    (c) low level of tetra-iodothyronine,
    (d) low level of tri-iodothyronine.

2   Which one of the following may be prescribed to relieve Mrs Thorn's excessive perspiration?
    (a) atropine sulphate,
    (b) sodium chloride,
    (c) propranolol,
    (d) frusemide.

3   Which of the following regimes would be most beneficial to Mrs Thorn?
    (a) mobilization within her capabilities,
    (b) gentle ambulation and diversional therapy,
    (c) bed rest to reduce her oxygen requirements,
    (d) allowed up for toilet purposes to reduce her embarrassment.

4   Which of the following responses is correct when Mrs Thorn questions her
    need for a high fluid intake? It will:
    (a) keep her cool,
    (b) keep her mouth moist,
    (c) prevent urinary tract infection,
    (d) aid excretion of metabolic waste.

5   Which one of the following diets would be most appropriate for Mrs
    Thorn?
    (a) high fibre, fluids and carbohydrate,
    (b) high protein, fats and carbohydrate,
    (c) high protein, vitamins and fluids,
    (d) high sodium, glucose and fibre.

Mrs Doris Barber   aged 62 years, is a widow and lives alone. She has a
good relationship with her daughter who lives next door and who visits every
day. Recently the daughter found her lying unconscious on the kitchen floor.
She has now been admitted to hospital and a diagnosis of myxoedemic coma
has been made.

1   Which of the following is the cause of Mrs Barber's coma?
    (a) hypothermia,
    (b) hypothymia,
    (c) hyperglycaemia,
    (d) hyperthyroidism.

2   Which of the following is the correct time to wait when recording Mrs
    Barber's rectal temperature?
    (a) 1 minute,
    (b) 2 minutes,
    (c) 3 minutes,
    (d) 4 minutes.

3   Which of the following may the nurse observe when Mrs Barber regains
    consciousness?
    (a) increased intolerance to heat,
    (b) diminished tolerance to noise,
    (c) diminished cognitive processes,
    (d) increased restlessness and irritability.

4   Which of the following is the most appropriate care for Mrs Barber's skin?
    (a) soap and water,
    (b) use of moisturizing cream,
    (c) application of talcum powder,
    (d) exposure to ultra violet light.

5   Which one of the following symptoms is Mrs Barber most likely to experience?
    (a) bruising,
    (b) delirium,
    (c) constipation,
    (d) irritability.

6   Which of the following will ensure that Mrs Barber receives her thyroxine therapy?
    (a) supervision by her daughter,
    (b) advise her to take it daily,
    (c) explain her condition to her,
    (d) daily visit from the district nurse.

Mrs Rosemary Kynaston   is 28 years old and her husband John is 32 years. They have been married for 7 years and have tried unsuccessfully to start a family. An appointment has been made for them by their doctor to see a gynaecologist at the local hospital out-patients department.

1   Which of the following is the time span after which Mr and Mrs Kynaston will be considered infertile?
    (a) 6 months,
    (b) 12 months,
    (c) 18 months,
    (d) 24 months.

2   Which of the following is necessary before the doctor examines Mrs Kynaston?
    (a) perineal toilet,
    (b) empty her bladder,
    (c) provide a specimen of urine,
    (d) discuss the method of contraception used.

3   Which of the following is normally the first step when investigating
    infertility?
    (a) post-coital test,
    (b) hysterosalpingogram,
    (c) seminal fluid analysis,
    (d) premenstrual endometrial biopsy.

4   Which of the following characteristics will indicate that Mrs Kynaston is
    ovulating? The ovulatory mucus is:
    (a) thin and scanty,
    (b) thick and cheesy,
    (c) clear and copious,
    (d) copious and white.

Mrs Anne Keene-Carey   is 52 years of age and has just been diagnosed as
having hyperparathyroidism.

1   With which one of the following problems will Mrs Keene-Carey present?
    (a) osteochondritis,
    (b) Heberden's nodes,
    (c) osteophytes in the joints,
    (d) decalcification of the bones.

2   Which one of the following is a complication of hyperparathyroidism?
    (a) brittle nails,
    (b) renal calculi,
    (c) cholelithiasis,
    (d) carpopedal spasm.

3   Which of the following foods will Mrs Keene-Carey be advised to avoid?
    (a) eggs,
    (b) liver,
    (c) peanuts,
    (d) tomatoes.

4   For which of the following reasons will Mrs Keene-Carey pass large
    volumes of urine? This is due to:
    (a) raised blood urea and creatinine,
    (b) raised serum glucose and potassium,
    (c) excretion of sodium and water by the kidney,
    (d) excessive amounts of calcium and phosphorus in the kidney.

Mr George Mellor   aged 43 years, is admitted to your ward with diabetes insipidus.

1   Which of the following is the cause of diabetes insipidus? The body's inability to secrete:
   (a) adrenocorticotrophic hormone,
   (b) antiduretic hormone,
   (c) cortisol,
   (d) insulin.

2   Which of the following are characteristic of diabetes insipidus?
   (a) anaemia, polyuria,
   (b) oliguria, anaemia,
   (c) polydipsia, oliguria,
   (d) polyuria, polydipsia.

3   Of which of the following symptoms may Mr Mellor have complained?
   (a) tiredness, muscular pains,
   (b) muscular pains, obesity,
   (c) constipation, tiredness,
   (d) obesity, constipation.

4   Which one of the following members of the health care team will be involved in the diagnosis of diabetes insipidus?
   (a) dentist,
   (b) urologist,
   (c) orthodontist,
   (d) ophthalmologist.

5   Which of the following should be carried out to aid diagnosis?
   (a) urogram, skull X-ray,
   (b) skull X-ray, visual fields,
   (c) electrocardiogram, urogram,
   (d) visual fields, electrocardiogram.

6   In which one of the following preparations will Mr Mellor receive vassopressin for the rest of his life? By:
   (a) intramuscular injection,
   (b) subcutaneous injection,
   (c) oral tablet,
   (d) nasal spray.

Ann Evans   is 28 years old and an insulin-dependent diabetic. She has been suffering from intermittent abdominal pain and is admitted to hospital for examination under anaesthetic and laparoscopy. This is her first anaesthetic and Ann is extremely anxious.

1   Which of the following is the most likely cause of Ann's glycosuria on the evening before her operation?
(a) stress,
(b) loss of appetite,
(c) change of routine,
(d) alteration in treatment.

2   Which of the following regimes will be prescribed for Ann on the morning of her operation? Nothing to eat or drink for:
(a) 6 hours before surgery,
(b) 8 hours before surgery,
(c) 6 hours before surgery and an infusion of dextrose,
(d) 8 hours before surgery and an infusion of dextrose.

3   Which one of the following is the prime observation made by the nurse when Ann returns from theatre? Ann's:
(a) pulse,
(b) breathing,
(c) urine output,
(d) infusion rate.

4   Which of the following actions should the nurse take when Ann seems confused and complains of a headache 8 hours after her operation?
(a) inform the doctor,
(b) perform urinalysis,
(c) give her a sweet drink,
(d) record her blood pressure.

5   Which of the following actions should the nurse take when she finds Ann asleep but sweating profusely?
(a) place a fan by her bed,
(b) record her temperature,
(c) wake her up immediately,
(d) remove some of the bedclothes.

Mr Edward French   aged 34 years, has been a diabetic for 20 years, and keeps in very good health. He has been admitted to your ward for removal of his wisdom teeth under general anaesthetic.

1   Which of the following would be used to control Mr French's diabetes during surgery?
(a) give insulin as usual,
(b) omit insulin the morning of surgery,
(c) intravenous infusion with added insulin,
(d) insulin on morning of surgery and oral glucose with premedication.

2   Which one of the following insulin preparations will be used in the immediate postoperative period to control his diabetes.
(a) lente,
(b) Actrapid,
(c) semi-lente,
(d) protamine zinc.

3   Which of the following is the correct time to start mouth washes post-operatively? After:
(a) 6 hours,
(b) 12 hours,
(c) 18 hours,
(d) 24 hours.

4   Which one of the following is the most appropriate mouthwash solution to use?
(a) cold bicarbonate,
(b) warm bicarbonate,
(c) cold saline,
(d) warm saline.

5   Which of the following should be used to monitor the state of Mr French's diabetes?
(a) six-hourly urinalysis,
(b) six-hourly B.M. Stix,
(c) daily urinalysis,
(d) daily B.M. Stix.

6   For which one of the following periods will Mr French have to take a course of prophylactic antibiotics?
(a) 3 days,

(b) 5 days,
(c) 7 days,
(d) 10 days.

Mr Alan Houseman   aged 34 years, has been admitted for repair of his right inguinal hernia. Alan has been a diabetic for the last 8 years and is well controlled on insulin. He is also a very keen badminton player.

1   Which of the following observations are important to record 6 hourly in the 24 hours before Alan's surgery?
(a) temperature, urinalysis, blood pressure,
(b) blood pressure, temperature, pulse,
(c) urinalysis, pulse, respiration,
(d) pulse, urinalyis, temperature.

2   Which one of the following is the most appropriate when Alan's insulin is due? The nurse should:
(a) offer to draw up the insulin for him,
(b) offer to give the injection for him,
(c) administer the injection herself,
(d) insist he gives it to himself.

3   Which of the following is Alan most likely to require preoperatively?
(a) infusion, physiotherapy,
(b) evacuant enema, infusion,
(c) physiotherapy, chest X-ray,
(d) chest X-ray, evacuant enema.

4   Which one of the following types of insulin is Alan most likely to have on the day of his operation?
(a) Actrapid,
(b) biphasic,
(c) isophane,
(d) zinc suspension.

5   Which of the following is the most appropriate response when Alan asks when he can play badminton again? After:
(a) 4 weeks,
(b) 8 weeks,
(c) 12 weeks,
(d) 16 weeks.

Jenny Miller   is a 32-year-old insulin-dependent diabetic who is recovering from ketoacidosis. She was admitted 12 hours ago, unconscious. Her condition resulted from gastroenteritis.

1   Which of the following is the prime reason for Jenny having a urethral catheter introduced on admission? To:
(a) prevent incontinence,
(b) test her urine for ketones,
(c) test her urine for glucose,
(d) measure her urine output hourly.

2   For which of the following reasons will Jenny have a nasogastric tube introduced on admission? To:
(a) provide glucose,
(b) prevent vomiting,
(c) provide nutrition,
(d) measure gastric secretions.

3   Which of the following is the effect of infection on a diabetic person?
(a) decreased carbohydrate requirement,
(b) increased carbohydrate requirement,
(c) decreased insulin requirement,
(d) increased insulin requirement.

4   For which of the following reasons will Jenny have been given insulin by the intravenous route?
(a) to utilize glucose rapidly,
(b) to convert blood glucose into glycogen,
(c) because fat breakdown should be stopped quickly,
(d) because subcutaneous insulin will be poorly absorbed.

5   For which of the following reasons will Jenny have been given intravenous dextrose when her blood glucose was approaching normal values? To:
(a) provide energy,
(b) replace fluid loss,
(c) avoid hypoglycaemia,
(d) replenish glycogen stores.

6   Which of the following should be the nurse's first action when Jenny regains consciousness?
(a) B.M. Stix test,
(b) record the time,
(c) inform the doctor,
(d) explain to her what has happened.

7   Which of the following instructions should Jenny be given when she asks
    what adjustment she could make to her insulin when she feels ill and
    unable to eat?
    (a) omit insulin until she feels like eating,
    (b) omit one dose of insulin,
    (c) reduce her insulin dose,
    (d) never omit her insulin.

8   Which of the following actions should Jenny be advised to take if she finds
    ketones in her urine?
    (a) increase her insulin dose,
    (b) reduce her fat intake,
    (c) drink extra fluid,
    (d) consult her doctor.

Mr Arthur Norris   is a 58-year-old married gentleman who manages his
own shoe shop. He has had a symptomless enlarged thyroid gland for many
years. Drug therapy has proved ineffective in reducing the size of the gland, so
2 days ago he underwent surgery for removal of a large adenoma on the left
lobe of the thyroid gland. His recovery has been uneventful until today when
he began to complain of pins and needles in his feet and numbness in his
fingers.

1   Which one of the following symptoms will indicate that Mr Norris was
    developing tetany? A:
    (a) hoarse voice,
    (b) weak hand grip,
    (c) high-pitched voice,
    (d) tremor of the hands.

2   Which one of the following is responsible for the development of Mr
    Norris' tetany?
    (a) hypercalcaemia,
    (b) hyperkalaemia,
    (c) hypocalcaemia,
    (d) hypokalaemia.

3   Which of the following is the main function of the parathyroid glands? To:
    (a) secrete the hormone calcitonin,
    (b) aid the deposition of calcium in bone,
    (c) maintain normal plasma calcium levels,
    (d) inhibit the deposition of calcium in the body.

4   Of which one of the following may Mr Norris also complain?
    (a) carpo-pedal spasm,
    (b) urinary retention,
    (c) blurred vision,
    (d) bronchospasm.

5   In which one of the following ways is Mr Norris' condition treated?
    Calcium gluconate by:
    (a) diluted intravenous injection,
    (b) bolus intravenous injection,
    (c) intramuscular injection,
    (d) subcutaneous injection.

6   Which of the following side effects may Mr Norris experience after this
    treatment?
    (a) renal colic,
    (b) hyperventilation,
    (c) thrombophlebitis,
    (d) cardiac arrhythmias.

Miss Gwen Slade   a 28-year-old home economics teacher, has found it
increasingly difficult to grip her cooking utensils due to discomfort in her
wrists and hands. She consulted her doctor who has referred her to the local
endocrinologist because he suspects she may have acromegaly.

1   Which of the following signs would have lead her doctor to suspect
    acromegaly?
    (a) prominent brows, buffalo lump, large feet,
    (b) deep voice, large hands, prominent brows,
    (c) large feet, buffalo lump, exophthalmos,
    (d) large hands, exophthalmos, deep voice.

2   Which of the following causes acromegaly? Excessive secretion of:
    (a) oxytocin,
    (b) aldosterone,
    (c) vasopressin,
    (d) somatotrophin.

3   Which of the following symptoms may Miss Slade mention during the
    admission interview?
    (a) amenorrhoea, visual disturbances,
    (b) menorrhagia, visual disturbances,

   (c) amenorrhoea, oliguria,
   (d) menorrhagia, oliguria.

4   Which one of the following is likely to be found during routine urinalysis
    after Miss Slade has been admitted?
    (a) glycosuria,
    (b) haematuria,
    (c) proteinuria,
    (d) urobilinogen.

5   Which of the following responses is the most appropriate when Miss Slade
    asks why she is having a chest X-ray?
    (a) it is performed routinely,
    (b) in case she has surgery,
    (c) to check lung fields,
    (d) to assess heart size.

6   Which of the following are important to note during Miss Slade's
    admission?
    (a) hypotension, tachycardia,
    (b) hypotension, bradycardia,
    (c) hypertension, tachycardia,
    (d) hypertension, bradycardia.

Mrs Jean McCleod   aged 43 years, is happily married with two sons aged
11 and 14 years. Twelve months ago she discovered a lump in her right breast
which her GP diagnosed as a benign adenoma. Recently she visited her doctor
again complaining of severe back pain. He has arranged her immediate
admission to hospital for investigations of carcinoma of the breast, biopsy of
the lump and possible right mastectomy.

1   Of which of the following symptoms may Mrs McCleod also complain?
    (a) an area of erythema on the right breast,
    (b) skin discolouration of the right breast,
    (c) a painful lump in the right axilla,
    (d) asymmetrical breasts.

2   Which of the following questions is particularly relevant to Mrs
    McCleod's condition?
    (a) 'Do you smoke?',
    (b) 'How did you feed your babies?',

(c) 'Have you ever had trauma to your breasts?',
(d) 'What methods of contraception do you use?',

3   Which one of the following will be performed to investigate Mrs McCleod's back pain?
(a) myelogram,
(b) bone scan,
(c) spinal X-rays,
(d) intravenous urogram.

4   In which of the following ways may Mrs McCleod be best supported throughout the preoperative period? By:
(a) safe and efficient physical preparation for surgery,
(b) being allowed time to express her fears and anxieties,
(c) inclusion of her husband in discussion of her condition,
(d) complete honesty from all members of the health care team.

5   For which of the following will Mrs McCleod's blood be tested? To determine her blood group and:
(a) acid phosphatase and haemoglobin,
(b) acid phosphatase and clotting time,
(c) alkaline phosphatase and haemoglobin,
(d) alkaline phosphatase and clotting time.

6   Which of the following would be most appropriate for the nurse to perform prior to surgery?
(a) mark the affected breast and shave the right axilla and breast,
(b) shave the right side from mid-line front to mid-line back, clavicle to umbilicus,
(c) shave the right breast and axilla and clean the area in a Savlon bath,
(d) supervise Mrs McCleod while she shaves and washes her right breast and axilla.

Margaret Grantham   is a 68-year-old widow who was found to have diabetes mellitus during her menopause. It was well controlled with diet and chlorpropamide, but she has recently gained weight and is found to have glycosuria. She wears spectacles to correct myopia but complains of having blurred vision recently.

1   Which one of the following describes Mrs Grantham's diabetes?
(a) latent,
(b) brittle,

(c) maturity onset,
(d) secondary onset.

2   Which of the following will be found when Mrs Grantham's urine is tested?
(a) pale colour with low specific gravity,
(b) dark colour with low specific gravity,
(c) pale colour with high specific gravity,
(d) dark colour with high specific gravity.

3   Which of the following is the reason for Mrs Grantham's increased urine output? The osmotic effect of glucose in the:
(a) glomerulus,
(b) distal tubule,
(c) proximal tubule,
(d) Bowman's capsule.

4   Which one of the following is the most likely cause of Mrs Grantham's blurred vision?
(a) glaucoma,
(b) cataracts,
(c) retinopathy,
(d) lens distortion.

5   Which of the following describes the action of chlorpropamide? It:
(a) is oral insulin,
(b) converts glycogen into glucose,
(c) reduces insulin requirements,
(d) stimulates insulin production.

6   Which of the following will indicate Mrs Grantham's understanding of her diet? The nurse should:
(a) assess her eating habits,
(b) assess her knowledge of nutrition,
(c) record her pattern of carbohydrate intake,
(d) record her total daily carbohydrate intake.

7   Which one of the following should Mrs Grantham be advised to avoid while she is having a weight-reducing diet?
(a) apples,
(b) grapes,
(c) melons,
(d) oranges.

8   Which one of the following must the nurse consider when advising Mrs
    Grantham about her diet? Her:
    (a) obesity,
    (b) income,
    (c) activities,
    (d) preferences.

9   Which of the following is the appropriate response when Mrs Grantham
    asks if she should have her spectacles changed?
    (a) ask the doctor to examine her eyes,
    (b) ask the doctor to assess her vision,
    (c) have her eyes tested in about 6 weeks,
    (d) have her eyes tested as soon as possible.

Mr Arthur Edwards   aged 46 years, had a partial thyroidectomy
performed 5 days ago. He has experienced increased neuromuscular
excitability and tetany and this is thought to be caused by interference with
the blood supply to the parathyroid glands. Calcium gluconate (10%) was
given intravenously and now he is taking a calcium supplement orally.

1   Which of the following problems will Mr Edwards have experienced?
    (a) muscle cramps, bone pain, vomiting,
    (b) dysphagia, carpopedal spasm, bone pain,
    (c) carpopedal spasm, vomiting, muscle cramps,
    (d) dysphagia, muscle cramps, carpopedal spasm.

2   Which one of the following vitamins may be prescribed for Mr Edwards to
    aid the absorption of calcium?
    (a) A,
    (b) B,
    (c) C,
    (d) D.

3   Which one of the following medications may be prescribed for Mr
    Edwards?
    (a) magnesium trisilicate,
    (b) aluminium hydroxide,
    (c) sodium bicarbonate,
    (d) potassium iodide.

4   Which one of the following foods will Mr Edwards be asked to limit in
    order to avoid future complications?

(a) flour,
(b) butter,
(c) oranges,
(d) carrots.

5   Of which of the following problems may Mr Edwards complain if the parathormone deficiency is prolonged?
(a) brittle nails, anorexia, thin hair,
(b) anorexia, constipation, coarse skin,
(c) thin hair, coarse skin, brittle nails,
(d) coarse skin, brittle nails, constipation.

6   Which of the following will Mr Edwards be advised to do?
(a) avoid alcohol,
(b) take extra fluids,
(c) take more exercise,
(d) avoid lifting heavy objects.

Elizabeth Page   is 26 years old and has recently been made redundant after working in a factory since she left school. She was diagnosed as having primary adrenal insufficiency, which is being treated with steroid therapy, since when has kept her in good health. Now she has abdominal pain with diarrhoea and vomiting; because of her weak and rapidly deteriorating condition, a neighbour takes her to the Accident and Emergency Department at the local hospital.

1   Which of the following disorders is the most likely cause of Elizabeth's symptoms?
(a) acute anxiety,
(b) gastroenteritis,
(c) acute glomerulonephritis,
(d) acute corticoid insufficiency.

2   Which one of the following is the most likely reason for Elizabeth's illness?
(a) anxiety,
(b) dieting,
(c) pyrexia,
(d) infection.

3   Which of the following will occur if Elizabeth is not treated immediately? Severe:

(a) hypertension and oedema,
(b) hypotension and jaundice,
(c) haematemesis and melaena,
(d) hypoglycaemia and dehydration.

4   Which of the following treatments will be administered intravenously immediately?
(a) normal saline, aldosterone,
(b) dextran, potassium, glucagon,
(c) dextrose, potassium, antibiotic,
(d) dextrose saline, hydrocortisone.

5   In which one of the following positions will Elizabeth be nursed in bed?
(a) Fowlers,
(b) recumbent,
(c) semi-prone,
(d) orthopnoeic.

ANSWERS

Mrs Margaret James

1 (d) Only correct answer.
2 (a) Feelings of depression at this age are most often associated with social events, e.g. family grown up and left home.
3 (b) Only practical advice to reduce vasodilation.
4 (d) Decreased female hormones reduce vaginal secretions.
5 (a) Is the only answer that encourages her to examine her symptoms and identify the reasons for them.
6 (d) Only correct answer.
7 (c) A counsellor enables an individual to cope with situations that cannot be changed.

8 (b) Loss of oestrogens causes skeletal decalcification.

David Sutton

1 (b) Fibre enables glucose to be absorbed slowly from the intestine so maintaining a more normal blood sugar level.
2 (c) Fibrosis interferes with the absorption of subcutaneous insulin.
3 (b) A diabetic is prone to athero-sclerosis and infection and unnecessary trauma to the periphery should be avoided.
4 (b) All the others contain sugar.
5 (a) Only correct answer.

Mrs Prudence Whittaker

1 (c) The only combination associated with maturity onset diabetes.

2 (c) People are more likely to co-operate if they understand the reasons for their management.

3 (d) The only one that will be able to provide practical help and advice in the day-to-day management of her diabetes.

4 (b) The only correct answer.

Mr Maurice Kenney

1 (a) Deposition of atheroma causes narrowing of the lumen resulting in ischaemia.

2 (d) Incision needs to be made above the level of arterial damage to ensure adequate blood supply for healing.

3 (a) Rehabilitation has to start before surgery.

4 (b) Knowing his centre of gravity enables him to be mobile.

Mrs Jennings

1 (c) Only recipient for blood group AB.

2 (b) Owing to postoperative position in the event of haemorrhage blood trickles to the nape of the neck.

3 (b) Bleeding into the tissues causes pressure on the trachea and will be the first complaint of the patient.

4 (b) Pressure on the trachea causes dyspnoea; see previous question.

5 (a) The most likely cause is haemorrhage, removal of skin clips allows blood to escape thereby relieving pressure on the trachea.

6 (d) Haemorrhage may occur as blood pressure returns to normal limits and dislodges a clot or loosely applied ligature.

Mrs Emma Blake

1 (b) Steroids act as an antagonist to insulin.

2 (d) Steroids are known gastric irritants.

3 (c) Steroids cause decalcification of bone.

4 (a) Electrolysis is permanent treatment.

5 (d) Reduced resistance to infection when taking steroids.

Debbie Frances

1 (c) Only correct answer.

2 (d) Preoperative assessment is necessary in case of damage to the recurrent laryngeal nerves during surgery.

3 (a) Hyperpyrexia is a sign of thyroid crisis.

4 (a) Healing is rapid at this site.

5 (d) The hoarse voice caused by the endotracheal tube usually settles by the fourth day.

6 (b) To prevent contraction of the scar.

7 (b) Most honest answer. The scar blends with the natural contours of the neck.

Mr Ross

1 (d) Ulcers heal by second intention of which granulation and fibrosis is a part.

2 (c) Diabetics are prone to peripheral neuropathy and testing with the elbows gives an accurate assessment of water temperature.

3 (d) Burns may result due to peripheral neuropathy.

4 (d) Due to peripheral neuropathy.

5 (a) Results in uneven pressure on the soles of the feet.

6 (b) The least traumatic measure.

7 (d) Involves use and inspection so only practical answer.

Mrs Julia Craven

1 (c) The side room enables all her needs to be met.

2 (b) Only correct combination. Amenorrhoea caused by hormone imbalance, sweating and palpitations due to a raised metabolic rate.

3 (a) Only correct answer.

4 (d) The only nonstimulant.

5 (d) Thyrotoxicosis is associated with severe weight loss.

6 (b) Increased pulse rate will result from an increased demand for oxygen.

7 (b) Only correct answer.

Constance Smith

1 (a) Only correct combination. Gluconeogenesis causes loss of limb muscle, facial plethora due to skin atrophy, and central obesity due to fluid retention.

2 (b) Only correct combination. Bruising due to capillary fragility, acne due to increased adrenal androgens and striae due to stretching of the skin.

3 (a) Excessive androgens causes virilism.

4 (b) A simple, general assessment of skeletal muscle function.

5 (a) Potassium is necessary for normal muscle function.

6 (d) Sodium retention causes increased circulating volume.

Miss Evelyn Gladwell

1 (a) Caused by decreased metabolism.

2 (b) Only correct combination. Thyroid hormones are

necessary for healthy skin
and hair and maintaining
metabolic rate.
3 (b) Lowered metabolism reduces
core temperature.
4 (d) Deposition of mucopoly-
saccharide causes nerve
compression.
5 (a) Replacement therapy is
essential for a normal
metabolism.
6 (a) See question 5.

Mrs Ruth Coates

1 (c) This diet counteracts gluconeogenesis.
2 (a) To replace excessive loss of
potassium.
3 (c) Adrenal hormones are no
longer available to play their
role in the maintenance of
blood pressure.
4 (a) Only correct combination in
the light of adrenalectomy.
5 (b) To prevent postural
hypotension.

Mrs Reeves

1 (b) Only correct answer from
available statistics.
2 (a) Only correct answer.
3 (b) This position will allow both
venous and lymphatic
drainage.
4 (d) Stretching deprives the
wound edges of blood supply
and necrosis occurs.

5 (d) A bra that Mrs Reeves has
used before is less likely to
cause discomfort.
6 (a) The most truthful answer.

Jennifer and Tim Mills

1 (c) Most commonly accepted
definition.
2 (c) Disordered ovulation is
commonest cause of female
infertility, twice as common
as a male factor.
3 (c) This is an indicator of luteal
function and is considered
the most satisfactory index of
ovulation.
4 (a) Only practical method of
obtaining a complete sample.
5 (a) Ovulation occurs mid-cycle.
6 (d) Is the kindest way to help
them accept the reality of the
present situation.

Mrs Mary West

1 (b) Only correct combination of
features resulting from
thyroid crisis.
2 (d) Chlorpromazine has sedative
and antipyretic properties.
3 (b) Glucose is required to meet
the extra energy demand pro-
duced by increased metabolism.
4 (d) Potassium iodide given intravenously should rapidly
counteract the effect of the
circulating thyroxine.

Mark Springer

1 (b) Immediate action must be taken to raise his blood sugar.
2 (a) Only correct answer.
3 (d) Alcohol inhibits the conversion of glycogen into glucose in the liver.
4 (a) Experiential learning.
5 (c) Adrenaline output is increased in an effort to raise blood glucose.

Gareth Morgan

1 (b) The only correct answer.
2 (a) Before teaching him anything, his level of knowledge about his own body needs to be ascertained and built on.
3 (d) A 15-year-old school boy is still growing.
4 (a) Abnormal fluctuation of blood sugar would not be detected whilst asleep.
5 (d) Fat necrosis is caused by giving injection in same site therefore reducing absorption.
6 (b) Chemicals in the tablet are caustic.
7 (c) Necessary to cope with energy expenditure.

Mr John Wellington

1 (a) Only correct answer.
2 (a) Only correct combination- headache caused by enlargement in skull, bitemporal hemianopia caused by enlarged pituitary pressure on optic chiasma and paraesthesia caused by pressure on median nerve.
3 (a) Only correct answer.
4 (a) Removal of pituitary ensures no release of adrenocorticot- rophin hormone (ACTH, corticotropin) to stimulate adrenal cortex, therefore hydrocortisone must be given to enable his body to react to the physiological stress of the surgery.
5 (a) Only correct combination- blood pressure gives a guide to effective steroid cover, nasal discharge could indicate a cerebrospinal fluid leak and excess urine output indicates diabetes insipidus.
6 (c) Only correct answer because there is no longer any anti- diuretic hormone (ADH, vasopressin) to control concentration.

Mr Victor Bussolino

1 (c) Dry gangrene is simply necrosis without any infection.
2 (d) A complication of diabetes is retinopathy.
3 (a) Enables him to maintain independence and self-esteem for as long as possible.

4 (d) Necrosed area should be left dry. Constrictive bandages would further reduce arterial blood supply.

5 (c) Keeping the foot cool will cause peripheral vasoconstriction, diverting blood supply to deep tissues thereby reducing pain. If the foot is dependent more efficient arterial blood supply is ensured.

6 (b) Only correct answer.

7 (d) Inadequate diabetic control will cause increased lipidaemia which in turn predisposes to atherosclerosis.

8 (b) Angiography will demonstrate the level of patency of the arteries and therefore this will determine level of amputation.

9 (d) Atherosclerosis causes hypertension which is a common complication of diabetes.

Miss Rita Walsh

1 (c) Only correct combination. Weight loss and tiredness caused by inability to convert glycogen into glucose. Areas of pigmentation are a common manifestation of unknown aetiology.

2 (d) Cortisone is necessary to combat physiological stress, therefore any infection may be overwhelming.

3 (d) Reduces exposure to infection- see previous question.

4 (b) Lack of cortisone causes hypotension.

5 (a) Lack of cortisone causes hypotension.

6 (d) Skin pigmentation is irreversible and this is positive and constructive advice.

7 (b) Caused by lack of aldosterone and cortisone production.

8 (d) Chemotherapy means replacement therapy.

Mrs Sylvia Thorn

1 (b) Serum level of tri-iodothyronine is always raised in thyrotoxicosis.

2 (c) Beta-blocking drugs block the response of ß-adrenoceptors to sympathetic stimuli.

3 (b) Mrs Thorn will not be receptive to enforced rest, but her hyperactivity can be regulated by diversional therapy.

4 (d) High metabolic rate produces excessive waste products.

5 (b) Calorie intake must equal energy expenditure.

Mrs Doris Barber

1 (a) Due to low metabolic rate.

2 (b) Only correct response.

3 (c) Depressed mental activity due to low levels of circulating thyroid hormone.

4 (b) Myxoedema is characterized by extremely dry skin and a moisturizing cream will help replace the moisture content.

5 (c) Low metabolic rate causing decreased peristalsis which predisposes to constipation.

6 (a) Reduced cerebral activity due to low levels of circulating thyroid hormones may cause her to forget her tablet. Her daughter, who is living next door, is the most appropriate person to oversee medication.

Mrs Rosemary Kynaston

1 (b) Most commonly accepted definition.

2 (b) Full bladder would inhibit bimanual palpation of uterus.

3 (c) Examination of seminal fluid is the easiest test to perform for infertility and therefore a logical starting point.

4 (d) At ovulation composition of cervical mucus alters to allow easier penetration by the spermatazoa.

Mrs Anne Keene-Carey

1 (d) High serum parathormone is responsible for the decalcification of bone.

2 (b) High serum calcium predisposes to formation of renal calculi.

3 (a) Only one containing calcium.

4 (d) Calcium and phosphorus are hydroscopic and therefore increase urine output.

Mr George Mellor

1 (b) Only correct answer.

2 (d) Polyuria results from the absence of antidiuretic hormone causing dehydration and extreme thirst.

3 (a) Dehydration results in loss of potassium.

4 (d) Enlargement of the pituitary causes pressure on the optic chiasma and disturbances in the visual fields.

5 (b) Skull X-ray will demonstrate an enlarged pituitary fossa. (see answer to question 4.)

6 (d) Readily absorbed by the nasal mucosa and preferable to injection.

Ann Evans

1 (a) Stress causes increased production of cortisol and adrenaline which convert glycogen into glucose thus raising serum glucose, resulting in glycosuria.

2 (c) Stomach contents will have passed into the duodenum in 6 hours and dextrose will prevent hypoglycaemia.

3 (b) All other observations are irrelevant unless the patient is breathing.

4 (c) Confusion and headache are signs of hypoglycaemia.

5 (c) Sweating is a sign of hypoglycaemia therefore Ann must be roused.

Mr Edward French

1 (c) Continuous infusion of insulin is necessary to deal with the stress of surgery. (see question 1 in the previous story.)

2 (b) Its rapid action ensures greater control of his diabetes.

3 (d) Twenty four hours ensures a secure clot reducing the risks of haemorrhage and socket infection.

4 (d) A warm physiological fluid is soothing and cleansing.

5 (a) It is the preferred assessment of diabetic control which causes no trauma to the patient.

6 (b) Five days is the standard length of time for prophylactic treatment.

Mr Alan Houseman

1 (a) Observation for infection, glycosuria and hypertension.

2 (b) It gives the patient an opportunity to rest the sites he normally uses for his injections.

3 (b) Bowel surgery requires an empty rectum and infusion will enable control of his diabetes.

4 (a) Its rapid action ensures greater control of his diabetes.

5 (b) A healthy young adult whose diabetes is well controlled should be able to resume his normal activities in 8 weeks.

Jenny Miller

1 (d) Jenny's condition causes shock and her renal function should be monitored.

2 (b) Ketoacidosis causes vomiting which must be prevented in case of inhalation.

3 (d) Infection increases metabolism, and more insulin is required to meet the increased demand for energy.

4 (d) Delayed absorption is caused by peripheral vasoconstriction due to the dehydration.

5 (c) The large doses of insulin given to treat hyperglycaemia may result in hypoglycaemia.

6 (d) The only answer that will meet Jenny's immediate need.

7 (d) Only correct answer.

8 (d) Ketonuria requires medical intervention.

Mr Arthur Norris

1 (c) High-pitched voice results from laryngeal spasm which is an early sign of tetany.

2 (c) The only correct answer.

3 (c) Secretion of parathormone which controls calcium levels.

4 (a) Increased excitability of nerves due to reduced serum calcium causes muscle spasm.

5 (a) Undiluted calcium gluconate causes cardiac arrhythmias.

6 (d) See previous question.

Miss Gwen Slade

1 (b) Only combination which results from excessive growth.

2 (d) Only correct answer.

3 (a) Amenorrhoea due to disturbed pituitary function. Visual disturbance due to enlargement of pituitary.

4 (a) Excessive somatotropin causes disturbance in glucose metabolism.

5 (d) Cardiac hypertrophy is associated with acromegaly.

6 (c) Thickening of the connective tissues results in increased peripheral resistance and hence hypertension. Tachycardia is a result of increased metabolism.

Mrs Jean McCleod

1 (d) Asymmetry of recent onset is indicative of carcinoma.

2 (b) Research indicates that mothers who breast feed their babies are less likely to develop carcinoma of the breast.

3 (b) Back pain is indicative of metastasis in this case and a bone scan will identify all bone metastases.

4 (c) Her husband is the most likely person to be able to provide the support she needs at this time.

5 (c) Alkaline phosphatase is increased in some malignant conditions and people with malignant disease are often anaemic.

6 (b) Correct skin preparation is the nurse's responsibility.

Margaret Grantham

1 (c) Diabetes occurring in middle age is known as maturity onset diabetes.

2 (c) Pale in colour as a result of polyuria and high sugar content raises specific gravity.

3 (b) Presence of glucose in the distal tubule will inhibit the reabsorption of water (glucose normally totally reabsorbed from proximal tubule).

4 (d) Lens distortion results from

the osmotic effects of glucose.

5 (d) Only correct answer.

6 (a) It is necessary to know what and when she eats to determine her understanding of her diet.

7 (b) Grapes have a high sugar content.

8 (b) Advice about diet must take into account the constraints of her income.

9 (c) Her lens' are most likely to have returned to normal in 6 weeks. (See question 4.)

Mr Arthur Edwards

1 (d) Symptoms of tetany — only correct combination.

2 (d) Only correct answer.

3 (b) Aluminium hydroxide binds with phosphorus in the intestine preventing its absorption.

4 (b) Butter contains phosphorus.

5 (c) Only correct combination resulting from parathormone deficiency.

6 (b) To promote excretion of phosphorus by the kidneys.

Elizabeth Page

1 (d) Only correct answer.

2 (a) Because of her adrenal insufficiency she is unable to respond to abnormal stresses.

3 (d) Blood glucose levels cannot be maintained and reabsorption of sodium is diminished in the kidney resulting in loss of water.

4 (d) See previous question.

5 (b) The most suitable position for a person with hypotension.